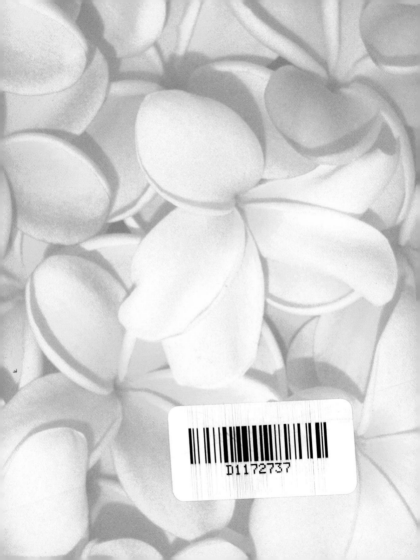

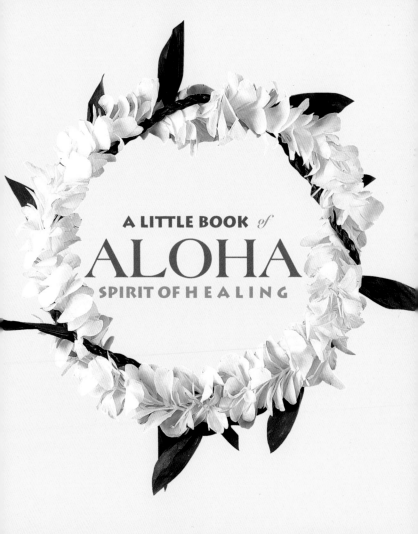

A LITTLE BOOK *of*

ALOHA

SPIRIT OF HEALING

Author's Note:
The information published has been
collected through interviewing people and healers
in Hawai'i to reflect as accurately as possible the current
beliefs of Hawaiian culture, traditional medicine and
healing practices. It is not intended to misrepresent,
alter beliefs or offend, and full respect and
acknowledgment is given that beliefs may
differ among Hawaiian people.

This is not a book of medical advice.
It is not the intent to recommend specific treatments.
None of the treatments described should be used
without the supervision of a healer.

A LITTLE BOOK *of*
ALOHA
SPIRIT OF HEALING

Renata Provenzano

Mutual Publishing

Permission to reprint Hawaiian proverbs and sayings,
and their translations, is courtesy of the Bishop Museum
'Ōlelo No'eau Hawaiian Proverbs and Poetical Sayings by Mary
Kawena Pukui (Bishop Museum Press). Copyright 1983
Bernice Pauahi Bishop Museum.

Library of Congress Catalog Card Number: 2001096770
ISBN-10: 1-56647-592-9
ISBN-13: 978-1-56647-592-1

Sixth Printing, April 2009
Design by Jane Hopkins

Mutual Publishing, LLC
1215 Center Street, Suite 210 • Honolulu, Hawai'i 96816
Ph: (808) 732-1709 • Fax: (808) 734-4094
info@mutualpublishing.com • www.mutualpublishing.com
Printed in Korea

Mahalo nui loa to all Hawaiian
healers and keepers of wisdom for allowing
me to sift through the ashes of your memories
…for your heartfelt grace
…and for sharing your healing practices
so people around the world can remember
how to love…to heal…to breathe.

Mahalo also to the islands of Hawaiʻi and the
Hawaiian people for sifting through the ashes of
my dreams…and stirring them to breathe.

FOREWORD

I HOʻOLULU, HOʻOHUALEI ʻIA E KA MAKANI.

What lay still in the calm is stirred by the wind.
—Henry P. Judd

"When a person stirs the ashes of the past, be sure he knows what he is doing, otherwise the fire will burn him. When you are playing with the ashes you are doing it because of innocence, because you are learning. You let in the oxygen (develop an interest) and start a fire, and ask us to burn again. We are the ashes of the past, so you are going to oblige by writing this book.

There are three types of flame. Yellow—the heat is enough to burn rubbish; all people can see it. Blue—enough to melt steel. And white—you cannot see white heat, you can only feel its great intensity.

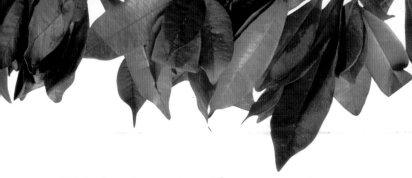

White heat is pure heat. If you are pure in your mind of what you want to do, then you will be on fire.

It only comes from nā akua (gods). Unseen but felt. If you ask and communicate with nā akua then you will experience white heat.

White heat is sacred. You do not use it all the time. That is what governs all people.

What you are writing is truth—that is good.

We see truth as a knowledge of things as they were, as they are, and as they are to come. "

—Levon Ohai, Lāʻau Lapaʻau
(Herbal Practitioner), Kauaʻi

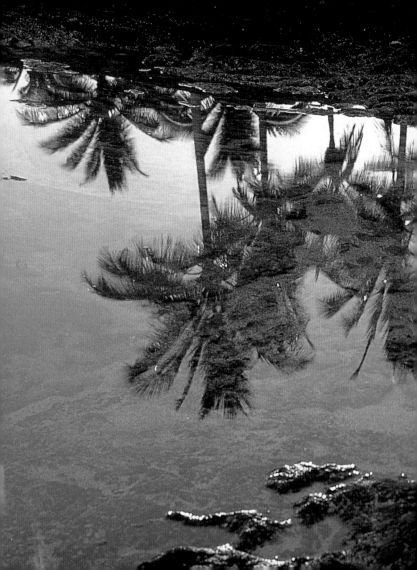

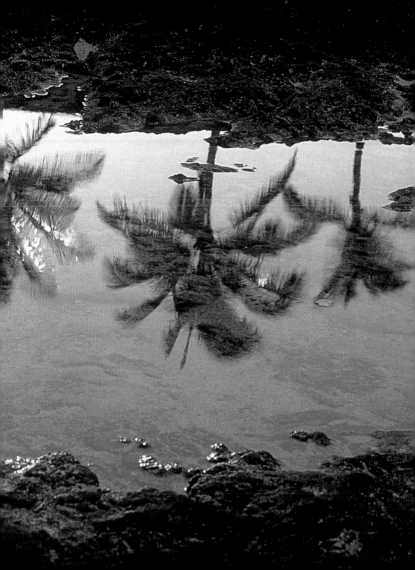

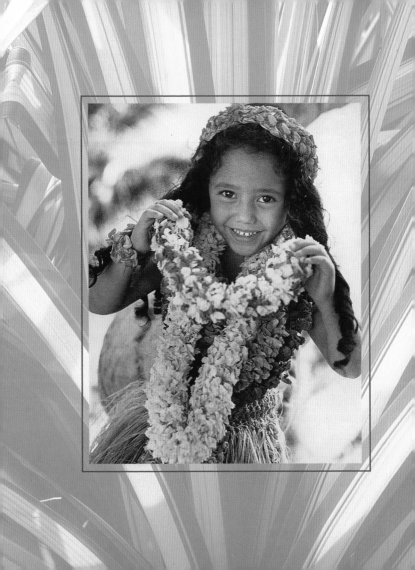

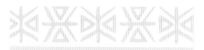

PREFACE

The popularity of *A Little Book of Aloha* has been an honor. I am thrilled so many people enjoyed learning about the Hawaiian spirit of aloha as much as I enjoyed writing about it. I am even more honored to know so many native Hawaiians have enjoyed the book as a memory of their grandparents' and ancestors' teachings in the form of ʻōlelo noʻeau (proverbs).

This second book, *A Little Book of Aloha: Spirit of Healing,* is a sacred gift from Hawaiian healers and keepers of wisdom across the islands as to how the spirit of aloha is in fact the key to Hawaiian well-being. Thousands of people around the world are drawn to the islands of Hawaiʻi every year to experience traditional healing—from massage and herbal medicines to physical and spiritual cleansing. They learn to tap into the mana (spiritual energy)

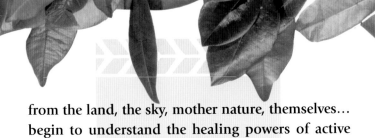

from the land, the sky, mother nature, themselves…
begin to understand the healing powers of active
volcano Kīlauea birthing every day…are renewed by
the graceful aloha of Hawaiian people that nourishes
their soul…and remember what their heart once knew.

A Little Book of Aloha: Spirit of Healing is the
current memory and thought on Hawaiian healing
as practiced hundreds of years past and today. Some
practice healing according to ancient beliefs pre-
Tahitian times, some incorporate modern deities and
religions, and some float in between. The common
thread is the spirit of aloha and aloha ʻāina (love of
the land) in order to come full circle with the earth
and the natural laws of life.

My kindest mahalo to my family, friends and
aloha angels all around the world for their support
and enthusiasm. A gracious mahalo to Linda

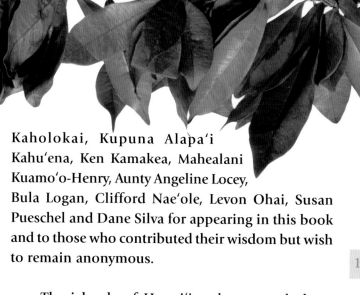

Kaholokai, Kupuna Alapaʻi
Kahuʻena, Ken Kamakea, Mahealani
Kuamoʻo-Henry, Aunty Angeline Locey,
Bula Logan, Clifford Naeʻole, Levon Ohai, Susan
Pueschel and Dane Silva for appearing in this book
and to those who contributed their wisdom but wish
to remain anonymous.

13

The islands of Hawaiʻi…where people have breathed the spirit of aloha for hundreds of years…they dance to please the gods…eat until they are tired…and dreams really do come true.

A culture so advanced…life is simple.

Aloha!
Renata Provenzano

The spirit of aloha is a way of life
and well-being embraced by native Hawaiians
for hundreds of years. Traditionally the word
aloha was a greeting reserved for loved ones by
first rubbing noses and then inhaling each other's
breath (*alo* = in the presence of, *hā* = breath of
life). To live with aloha is the secret to well-being
for the people of Hawai'i. It is an inner knowledge,
by birth, to be loving and genuine in all
interactions with people and nature, for all life is
connected. It is how you say hello, it is sharing
food, caring for strangers, a nod of the head,
understanding one another, a smile, kindness,
honesty, touch, empathy in times of grief and a
free willingness to love, as naturally as
children love...as naturally as mother
nature loves the earth.

14

HE PŪNĀWAI KAHE WALE KE ALOHA.

Love is a spring that flows freely.
—Mary Kawena Pukui

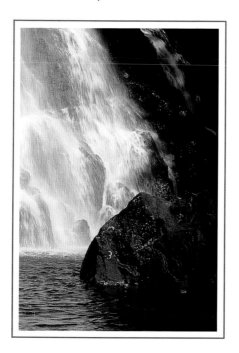

"The first medicine is forgiveness.
Before any one of us can heal ourselves we need to
have forgiveness. We need to have pono (balance).
If we cannot forgive ourselves, we cannot heal
others, we cannot heal anyone."

Kupuna Alapa'i Kahu'ena, Lā'au Lapa'au
(Herbal Practitioner), O'ahu

16

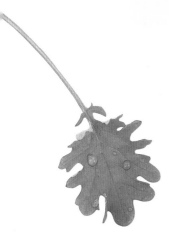

HOʻOKAHI NO LĀ'AU LAPAʻAU, O KA MIHI.

The first remedy is forgiveness.
—Kupuna Alapaʻi Kahuʻena

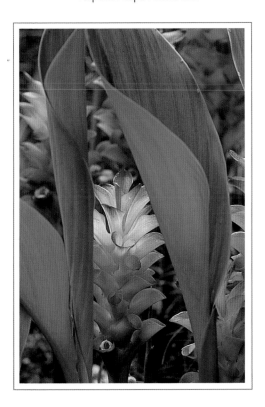

Hawaiians are renowned for their grace, good nature and happy disposition. Part of the many ways Hawaiians maintain their well-being is continual cleansing and being pono (in balance) with the world. To cleanse is to purify. One must purify the physical body as well as the mental, emotional and the spiritual. This is achieved through daily pule (prayer), forgiveness, massage, herbal medicine, fasting, going into the ocean and being one with nature. When people are very ill, some seek help from kāhuna (healers). To simply be still and ask nā akua (gods) to help is a divine intention to heal.

MAI KA PIKO O KE PO'O A KA POLI O KA WĀWAE, A LA'A MA NĀ KIHI 'EHĀ O KE KINO.

From the crown of the head to the soles of the feet,
and the four corners of the body.
—Mary Kawena Pukui

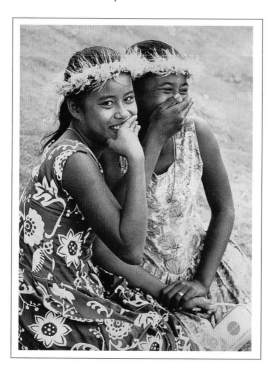

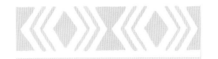

"Aloha has to begin with self.
You have to love yourself, you have to want
to heal yourself. Any aspect of dis-ease is a lack of
aloha. Aloha includes all the things aloha means,
there is all the respect. When you have respect you
start to heal. When you have lōkahi (peace or
unity) you start to heal. The answer is when you
look inside yourself—do you feel good about
yourself, are you secure of who you are, are
you aware you created everything you
wanted to create?"

Bula Logan, Lomilomi and Lāʻau Lapaʻau
(Herbal Practitioner), Oʻahu

OLA MAI ILOKO MAI.

Health comes from within.

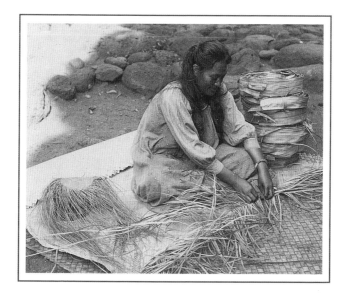

The innate relationship Hawaiians have
with the land is known as aloha ʻāina (love of the land)
—considered intrinsic to well-being.

"The ʻāina is where we go to get grounded.
That is what we base our aloha ʻāina on. We
manifest ourselves into everything that is physical
and that is how we get back in tune with the
spiritual. Humans are the only ones not in tune
with it. Where I am standing and where you are
standing *is* our closest spiritual world. At the
moment I am looking at the coastline, at coffee
trees, mango trees, banana trees. This place that I
love has been in the family 1,000 years and these
were all planted by my ancestors. It is recognized
as the mana, the spiritual self, caring. What they
nurture and I have gone into that realm. I know
the trees are all alive—it nurtures me, my
family, my children and whoever else."

Anonymous, Native Hawaiian Guide, Island of Hawaiʻi

UA MAU KE EA O KA ʻĀINA I KA PONO.

The life of the land is preserved in righteousness.
—Mary Kawena Pukui

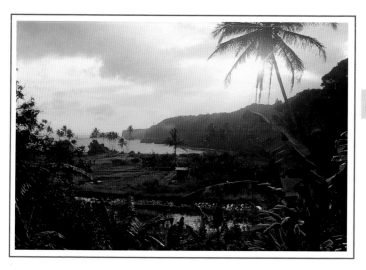

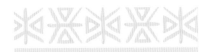

"Nature is one of our greatest healers.
There is healing in the wind, the sun, the moon,
the stars, the ocean, the stones, the songs of the
birds and the flowers. It is only for us to trust this
is so and allow ourselves to receive."

Linda Kaholokai, Island of Hawai'i

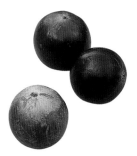

KA LĀ I KA MAULI OLA.

The sun at the source of life.
—Mary Kawena Pukui

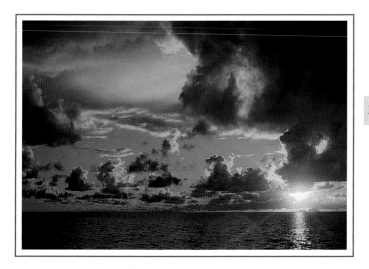

"When the heavens weep, the earth lives.
Sky father comes down to mother earth and to her
peaks. The mist is the sperm. So heavy rains come
from father and mother earth fruits. Everything
goes back to love, much love…love…love."

Kupuna Alapaʻi Kahuʻena, Lāʻau Lapaʻau
(Herbal Practitioner), Oʻahu

UWĒ KA LANI, OLA KA HONUA.

When the sky weeps, the earth lives.
—Mary Kawena Pukui

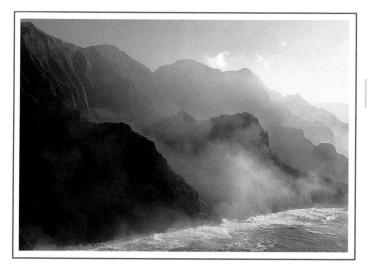

"Aloha ʻāina is total balance. The land
is significant because it holds our ancestors.
You must care for the provider, the land is the
provider. It gives you health and death, your food,
clothes, shelter and medicine. If you do not take
care of the ʻāina you are shooting yourself in the
foot. We need to think island—everything is finite,
sooner or later we will run out of something. In
days of old we took six fish, now we take 100 and
put it in the freezer so there is nothing left in the
ocean. We have become so accustomed to
moving fast and living life that we won't let
life live. The answers are right in front of
our eyes but we destroy it daily."

Clifford Naeʻole, Cultural Adviser, Maui

PŪʻALI KALO I KA WAI ʻOLE.

Taro, for lack of water, grows misshapen.
—Mary Kawena Pukui

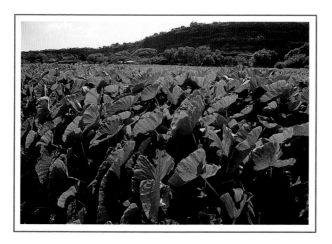

Most practitioners of herbal medicine, lomilomi massage, hula, chanting, ho'oponopono (making right more right) and other sacred healing acknowledge there are many different beliefs and practices because they were taught by different teachers and come from different islands. Some were taught by grandparents, aunties and uncles, or invited to learn by a kahuna (master). Mostly in Hawai'i healers are selected from a young age after having been observed by a kahuna. Students never ask to be taught. As healers their most important medicine is to be pono (in balance) themselves. To be pono, healers practice constant pule (prayer) and cleansing before, during and after healing people.

'A'OHE PAU KA 'IKE I KA HĀLAU HO'OKAHI.

All knowledge is not taught in the same school.
—Mary Kawena Pukui

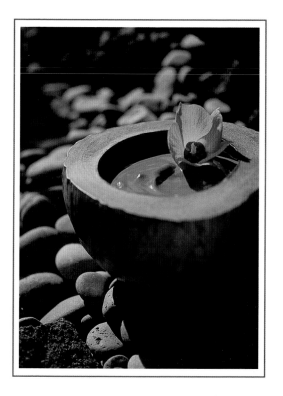

The early Polynesian voyagers brought
the ancient knowledge of herbal medicine
when they settled the Hawaiian Islands. Herbal
practitioners are known as kāhuna lāʻau lapaʻau
and the secrets of treating illness with herbs
(plants and flowers) have been passed down
through generations through storytelling and
tradition. Each practitioner may be taught
differently. Through their own intuition they learn
the tone of an herb and experiment with new
applications or use different parts of an herb for
healing. It is considered there are no such things
as weeds, just plants not yet understood…
just like people.

HE KEIKI ALOHA NĀ MEA KANU.

Beloved children are the plants.
—Mary Kawena Pukui

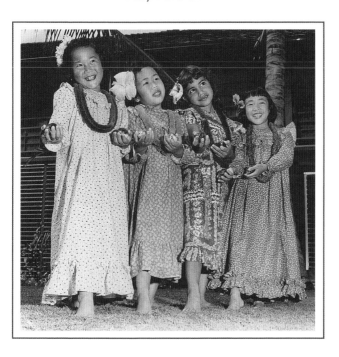

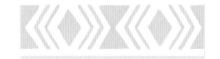

When administering herbal medicine,
a kahuna lāʻau lapaʻau (herbal practitioner) meets
with a sick person before choosing herbs, so
medicines are collected with that person in mind.
A sacred protocol is followed when gathering
medicines. First the plant is approached, told what
it will be used for and asked for its permission.
When guidance comes forth, a practitioner asks
the plant to be blessed for whoever needs it and
thanks akua. Once the herb is used it is never
thrown away as it carries the illness. It must be
dissolved physically and spiritually and
returned to the land or the ocean.

AIA KE OLA I KAHIKI.

Life is in Kahiki.
(Life and prosperity are in the care of the gods, and the gods are said to reside in Kahiki.)
—Mary Kawena Pukui

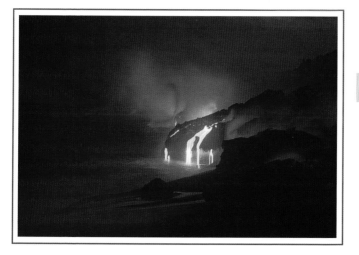

Popular Hawaiian herbs such as noni, 'awapuhi (ginger), kava, kīnehe (Spanish needle), kī (ti) and māmaki are prepared as teas and may be used to treat anything from diabetes to cleansing the digestive system, increasing energy or reducing phlegm. Others such as koali 'awa (morning glory) are pounded to make a poultice for wounds or broken bones and sometimes pa'akai (sea salt) or even a patient's mimi (urine) is mixed in to aid the herb's penetration.

OLA NŌ I KA PUA O KA ʻILIMA.

There is healing in the ʻilima blossoms.
(One of the first medicines given to babies. It is a mild laxative.)
—Mary Kawena Pukui

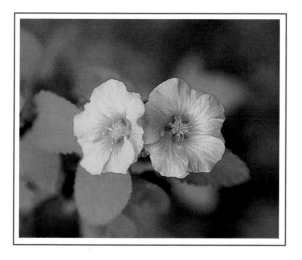

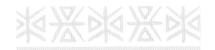

"My tūtū (grandfather) was an herbal
practitioner and he told me about the old
traditions and stories. I learned, one at a time,
where to get the herbs—what part of the mountain
or part of the ocean (dry, arid, wet areas). Herbs
are warriors. Warriors are very powerful and you
can always depend on them. They will fight for
you and if you know how to use them, they
will heal you. The belief of the Polynesians
is, when you use the herbs to go to battle,
they go to clean up."

Levon Ohai, Lā'au Lapa'au (Herbal Practitioner), Kaua'i

HE MAU KŪPUNA KOU, HE 'AI KO UKA, A HE I'A KO KAI. HE AHA KA INOA O KA PUA?

'AWAPUHI.

You have grandparents, food in the upland and
fish in the sea. What is the name of the flower?

Ginger blossom.
(Food in the upland is **'awa,** fish of the sea is **puhi.** The two words form **'awapuhi**.)
—Henry P. Judd

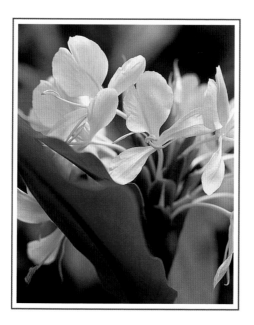

'Alaea is red dirt found only in certain areas of some islands. It is a powerful healer of conditions such as cancer, heart disease and diabetes. The rock is ground to a powder and usually mixed with 'ōlena (turmeric) and added to a small amount of water to drink. Today the 'alaea is used to dye T-shirts…and is in danger of running out.

KU'U 'UMEKE PĀKĀKĀ (HONUA).

My large calabash (earth).
(A calabash bowl is used for gifts to go in...the earth cradles all gifts.)
—Henry P. Judd

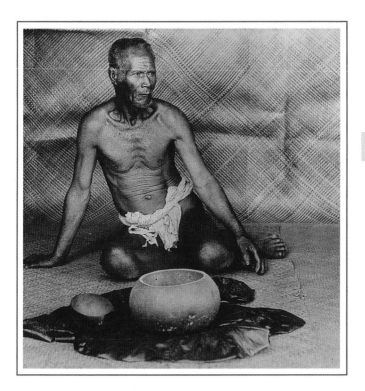

'Ōlena (turmeric) is known as a
miracle herb. It is a master and aids in healing
many ailments, particularly those related to
mucous and inflammation of the sinuses, ulcers,
lupus and sickness of the intestines. 'Ōlena may be
prepared as a drink to heal a weak bladder or
grated and strained for its juices as an eye wash
for glaucoma, near and far sightedness and
eyestrain. The most important step for the use of
all herbs is for it to be prepared in accordance
with protocol and blessed for the patient.

'ONO KĀHI 'AO LŪ'AU ME KE ALOHA PŪ KEKAHI.

A single roll of taro top is delicious if seasoned with affection.

(Not the gift, but how it is given.)

—Henry P. Judd

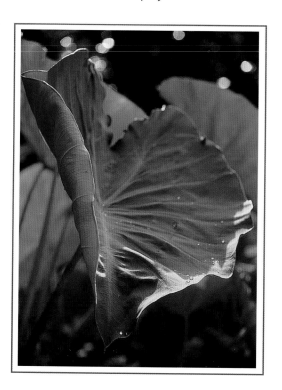

The taro plant is considered the
first Hawaiian. The evolution of the plant
stems from legend and today is a staple food in
Hawai'i, especially when pounded for making poi
(a thick paste to accompany meals). In days of
old, after the rains a kahuna lā'au lapa'au (herbal
practitioner) would capture the water pooled on
the leaves of the taro plants and use it for herbal
mixtures and healings. The taro plant is
sacred and a blessing from the gods.

(HAWAIIAN RIDDLE)

KUʻU WAHI IʻA	My little fish
MOKU KE POʻO	cut off the head
MOKU KA HIʻU	cut off the tail
HOʻIHOʻI I KA WAI	return to the water
A OLA HOU	it lives again
KE KALO	The Taro

—Henry P. Judd

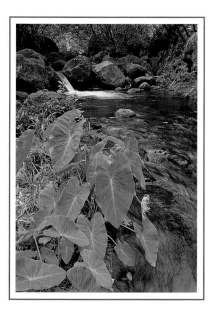

Hawaiians live in both worlds—
the visible and tangible on earth and
the spiritual, where their 'aumakua (family
spirit guides) reside. They gather information to
make life decisions from both the waking world
and in dreams, from signs, visitations, omens and
divine guidance. It is important to see beyond
what the eyes can see, listen for things that are not
said and recognize what your na'au
(gut instinct) already knows. Hawaiians are
naturally aware and connected to the spirit
and in being so create their life with pure
intention. They believe that life evolves as
nature intended and the right time will
come for all things.

'ANO LANI; 'ANO HONUA.

A heavenly nature; an earthly nature.
(Said of 'aumakua who make themselves visible to loved ones by assuming earthly form,
such as fish, fowl or animal, yet retain the nature of a god.)
—Mary Kawena Pukui

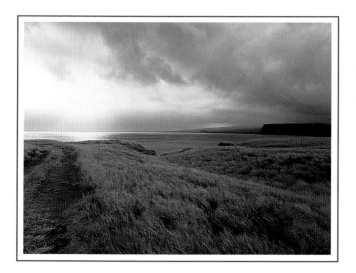

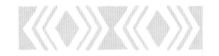

A lot of illness in the modern world
is caused by an obsession with competition and
acquisition. People ignore their inner desires and
cross boundaries with their own ethics in order to
work and feed themselves. It is difficult to pursue
your dreams and live the life you truly want to in a
society which demands financial success, but
Hawaiians believe if you really wish to pursue
something with the right intention, ke akua (god)
will bless you. Ke akua is able to move people,
change circumstances and make dreams come
true. A lomilomi healer I met in Oʻahu used to
work in his family's pizza business until he
decided he must pursue his gift to heal others. He
trusted in akua and soon enough he had a rent-
free room, received a massage table as a gift
and people arrived from all over the world
for his healing. If you pursue your passion—
that which you truly love—everything
else will fall into place.

NĀNĀ NĀ MOE.

Look to your dreams.

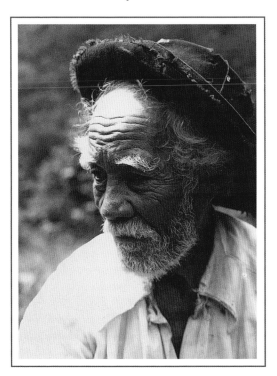

No medicine on earth will help you unless you are pono (in balance). In order to create pono the practice of ho'oponopono (making right more right) is important to healing. Pono is the balance between the physical and spiritual self and comes from within. When the mind and the heart disagree one must take the time to sit still and listen to the na'au (gut feeling) telling you what you have done right and what you have done wrong. Sometimes the wrongs you have committed towards other people or other energies may be things that are affecting you now.

The things you have done wrong, you need to make correct. Forgiveness brings power to you and to those who have wronged you. Further, if someone apologizes you must accept this and never speak of it again. If a grudge is held it becomes your kaumaha (burden) and will continue to make you ill.

LUHI ʻUʻA I KA ʻAI A KA LIO.

It is useless labor to get feed for the horse.
(It is a waste of labor to get medicine unless the sick has repented.)
—Henry P. Judd

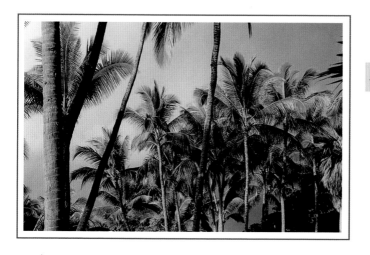

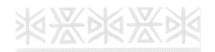

Cleansing the mind is an art
practiced daily for well-being and peace. In
the quiet of the evening, the day is reviewed. You
must forgive yourself and others. If you could have
interacted with someone more in keeping with
your soul, then you fix it in your thoughts. In
doing so you set the intention for a new pattern.
The blessing of a new day is the opportunity to set
a new intention. While not all of life's challenges
can be easily explained, Hawaiians believe there is
a reason for everything. That reason may even
come after the death of a person.

HE UKANA KO KA HOUPO.

A burden on the diaphragm.
(A problem in the mind.)
—Mary Kawena Pukui

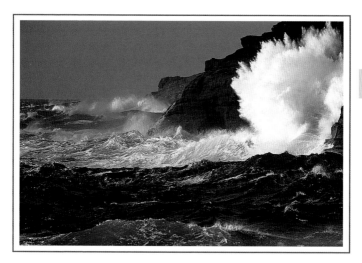

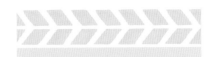

"In the Hawaiian culture, mind and body is never separate from spirit. Papa Henry Auwae (foremost Hawaiian herbal practitioner, now passed on) said 80% of healing is spiritually based and 20% is through using medicine or herbs. Quite often when you are ill you will be asked what is going on in the family, with relationships, in your heart or in your spirit."

Susan Pueschel, Bakken Foundation for the Five Mountains Community, Island of Hawai'i

54

E HOʻI KA WAʻA; MAI HOʻOPAʻA AKU I KA ʻINO.

**Make the canoe go back;
do not insist on heading into a storm.**
—Mary Kawena Pukui

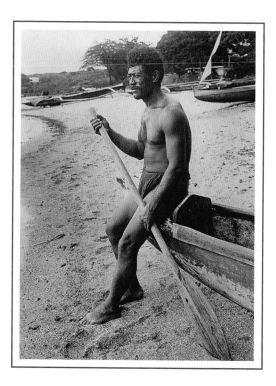

"Sometimes it is hard to fix a broken heart. It is the hardest thing to do. I have found practicing with the herbs, it is easy to heal a physical wound but to fix something that is in the heart and mind, it takes years sometimes. You really need to go by the spirit. You cannot pay money to heal an emotional thing."

Levon Ohai, Lāʻau Lapaʻau (Herbal Practitioner), Kauaʻi

56

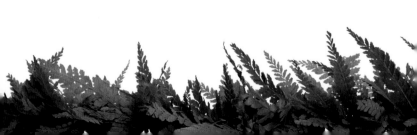

HAʻU KA MAKANI, HĀʻULE KE ONAONA, PILI I KA MAUʻU.

The wind blows, the scent is lost:
the perfume falls and stays close to the grass.
(Love is lost through anger, otherwise, love may fail but is easily recovered.)
—Henry P. Judd

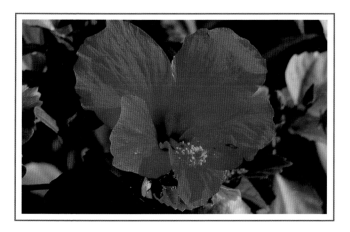

"Oki is a way of severing relationships
or patterns of the past. This ritual allows us to
disentangle ourselves from emotional links which
entrap us. We may choose to sever the energetic
connections with whomever or whatever is making
us ill or unhappy. Aka cords are the links between
us and the people and places we touch. To break
out of a pattern first you must deeply want to
create change. Then a personal reprogramming
begins and you create something new. This
process creates the image of the new pattern
and empowers it with focused spiritual
energy we call mana."

Dane Silva, Long Life Lomilomi Instructor and Practitioner,
Island of Hawai'i

E WĀHI KA MĀKĀHĀ I PI'I KA I'A.

Break the pond gate so the fish can get in.
(Break away from bad habits, then good can enter your life.)
—Henry P. Judd

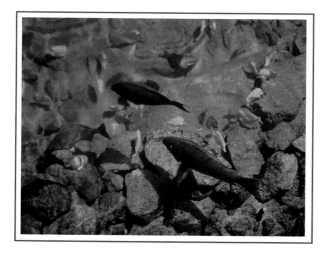

Hawaiʻi is home to surfing!
Surfing is a lifestyle, with surfers arranging
their work hours to ensure they can always catch
the best waves. The physical sport incorporates the
mind, spirit and the body...and the ultimate in
being pono (balanced)! Any surfer will tell you
they ride best when they ride *with* the wave
(nalu)...when they go with the situation, not
against it. It is important to remember that with
each new situation life brings, the nalu is
different. You will not always know what is
coming, as waves swell up from behind, so you
must position your board as best you
can...wait...then be ready
to surf with the nalu.

HE KĀʻEʻAʻEʻA PULU ʻOLE
NO KA HEʻE NALU.

An expert on the surfboard who does not get wet.
—Mary Kawena Pukui

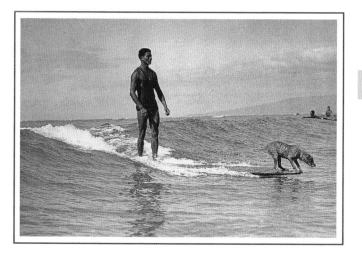

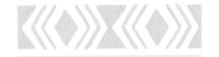

For some Hawaiians the honu
(turtle) represents the ʻaumakua (family
guardian spirit). Very similar to the word honu is
the word for earth—honua—and the turtle has
long been compared to the earth. The green turtle
in Hawaiʻi is one of the oldest animals and the
shape of the turtle's back perhaps resembled the
world as it was to Polynesians. Turtles are also
considered the ultimate navigators. They leave the
sands of their birth immediately after they dig
their way out of their incubators and may travel
800 miles from their birthplace, spend the next 20-
50 years of their lives elsewhere and then return to
the exact spot of sand of their births to mate and
nest. For the Polynesian navigator it was always
important to know your roots…know where you
came from…the sands of your birth…so
you could always find your way back home.

KA IʻA ʻAU MAI ME HE MANU.

The fish that swims with the movements of a bird.
(The turtle.)
—Mary Kawena Pukui

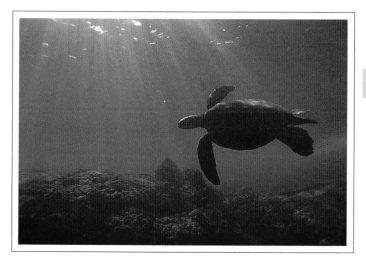

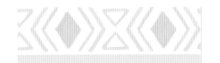

Before missionaries arrived, the melodic Hawaiian language was spoken, not written. In Hawaiian belief all words, as with all things, have mana (spiritual energy), so naming of people and places reflects powerful symbolism. Still today when children are born it may take up to a year for a child to be named as the name carries his or her destiny. People are taught to choose words with care as what you say becomes an intention and energy follows. Words can heal or destroy.

"I have been told by a Hawaiian spiritual master that the Big Island is a very powerful healing center for the world. It has to do with the name of this place: hā = breathe of life, wai = water of life; ī = divinity."

Susan Pueschel, Bakken Foundation for the Five Mountains Community, Big Island

I KA ʻŌLELO NO KE OLA, I KA ʻŌLELO NO KA MAKE.

Life is in speech, death is in speech.
—Mary Kawena Pukui

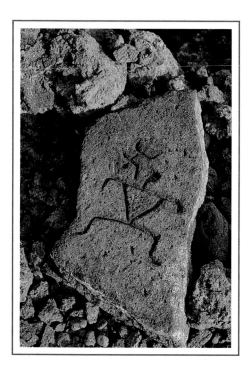

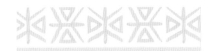

"The difference between the western
and the Hawaiian culture is that in the western
you need to see it before you can understand it. In
Hawai'i you just need to feel it. Sometimes you
need to believe in something before you can see it.
It is not imagination. I am a traditional healer and
practice old-style Hawaiian lomilomi called hā'hā.
We are trained to have eyes in all our fingers,
when they walk the body they find everything.
Every single one of us has this gift—we all have
the mana but it is the individual who has to bring
their energy up to par. Most of us are
gifted in what we do."

Ken Kamakea, Hawaiian Health Practitioner, Maui

HE ʻIKE PĀPĀLUA.

Dual knowledge.
(Gifted with second sight or extra perception)
—Mary Kawena Pukui

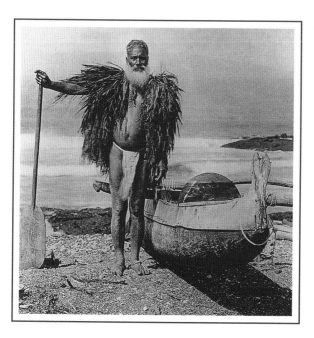

Massage and healing touch was never practiced for beauty and indulgence but as an essential step to cleanse and heal the body. Traditional lomilomi was not sensuous massage but a centuries-old sacred practice of chiropractic adjustments to reconnect and energize the body. Today lomilomi is mostly practiced as a deep tissue massage, with the practitioner often using elbows, even feet, to relax muscles and soothe pain. Healing stone massage uses heated lava rocks against the skin to increase circulation and draw out toxins. Laying of hands is similar to what westerners term reiki and has long been practiced throughout the islands. Kī (ti) leaf wraps help draw out fevers and heat from sunburn.

HE HALE KE KINO NO KA MANA'O.

The body is a house for the thoughts.
——Mary Kawena Pukui

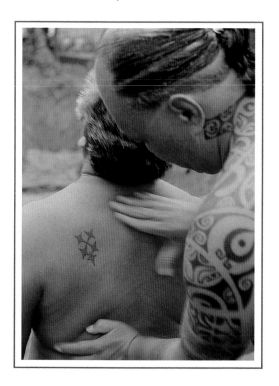

"This is the Moon Lodge. This is where women and young girls came during their menses, learned about their bodies, learned about taking care of themselves, learned to love their bodies. We had to overcome a lot of shame the missionaries' ideas put upon us. Our medicine was growing right around us. The mountains with the clay and sea salt from the ocean. You learn to heal your body and secrets of wellness: sharing loving massage, preparing them for life, for marriage, learning how to love the body (aloha kino), to give and receive pleasure from your own body. You can only do that if you are living in a well body."

Aunty Angeline Locey, Hawaiian Kupuna, Kaua'i

MANA I KA PUA UA MOHALA MĀLIE .

There is mana in the flower that has blossomed slowly.

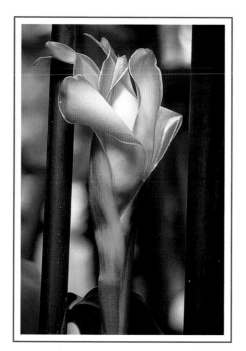

In Hawai'i beauty *is* living with aloha,
not an outwardly judgment of a person's body.
When Hawaiians use earth essences to cleanse and
adorn themselves—flowers in the hair, oils to
massage, salt scrubs to cleanse, leaves and flower
leis as adornments—it is never to cover or add to
themselves, but rather to become closer to and a
part of their environment...to be one with
nature...to have aloha 'āina.

E LEI KAU, E LEI HOʻOILO I KE ALOHA.

**Love is worn like a wreath through the summers
and the winters.**
—Mary Kawena Pukui

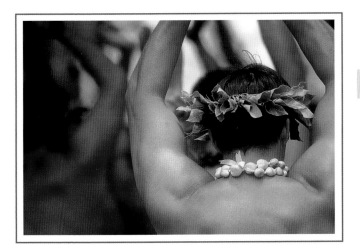

"Spiritually we are not complete if
we do not understand the responsibility we
carry for our bodies. Hula is a visual expression
of praise. The feet move from tropic to tropic
showing us not just space but place. Everything is
reflective of this universal order. Imagine if you
are standing above everyone, the movements are
forward going between the tropics, the stars and
the constellations. The connection happens when
it is done at sacred times (of the day or year). In
the old way, you would rise with the sun and
electrify your pikos (chakras)—look at the sun as
it comes out of the ocean and it would enlighten
and ignite us and give us strength."

Anonymous, Traditional Hula Practitioner, Kaua'i

HŌʻALEʻALE MĀNĀ I KE KAHA O KAUNALEWA.

Mānā ripples over the land of Kaunalewa.

(Said of movements of a dance. A play on ʻaleʻale [to ripple like water], referring to the hands, and lewa [to sway], referring to the movement of the hips.)

—Mary Kawena Pukui

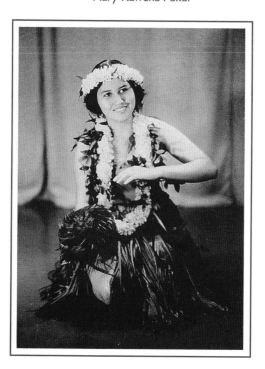

Family ('ohana) is not just
blood relatives, but all close friends are
considered 'ohana or calabash family. Hence the
title of aunty, uncle, cousin, sister or brother is
given to people who may not be direct family. In
an island culture, space is shared and so is life. It
is understood 'ohana is always there for each other
in times of need and in times of celebration.
This sense of 'ohana is extremely important
to Hawaiians for their sense of belonging, sense
of direction and sense of self. It is not
uncommon for Hawaiians to trace
their lineage back a thousand years.

E KOLO ANA NO KE ĒWE I KE ĒWE.

The rootlet will creep toward the rootlets.
(Of the same origin, kinfolk will seek and love each other.)
—Mary Kawena Pukui

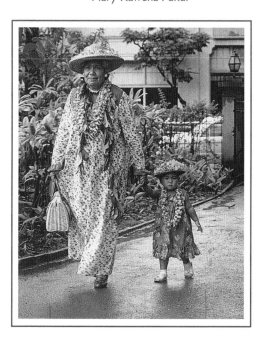

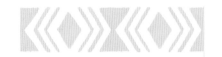

"For us, love is down to the depth
of the sea. Something that is serious, that is
born in the family. We are a family type of people.
Family is our solidarity, it is our government, it
goes back to time immemorial. Aloha means when
you give someone a lei, you do not buy the lei—
you make the lei with your own hands and
then you give it away and that lei is made
with love and respect and everything that
should be in the soul of man."

Levon Ohai, Lā'au Lapa'au (Herbal Practitioner), Kaua'i

AWAIĀULU KE ALOHA.

Love made fast by tying together (marriage).
—Mary Kawena Pukui

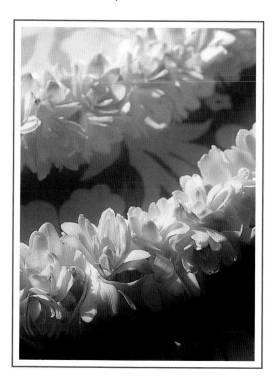

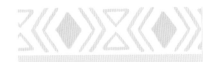

Keiki (children) carry the Hawaiian culture and traditions into the future. A child's first birthday is considered one of the most important and often celebrated with a lūʻau because in days of old many babies died in infancy. In a world so obsessed with power and so consumed with fear, it is easy to miss the simple pleasures in life. Be sure to remember the unconditional love of children. Listen to them tell the story of their day and how the little things excite and delight them. Watch how they invite everyone to play and make-believe. Hear the tinkle of their laughter come out loud from their belly and how they sing to their own tune. Children remind us of life, because they are all born with the knowledge of aloha.

HE LEI POINA ʻOLE KE KEIKI.

A lei never forgotten is the beloved child.
—Mary Kawena Pukui

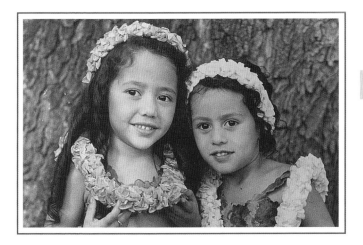

You will often hear in Hawai'i:
"we don't eat until we are full, we eat until we
are tired!" Food is a gift from the earth, so to
share food with family, at lū'au or with strangers
is sacred. The mana (spiritual energy) of the
land goes inside people to continue the
exchange of life energy.

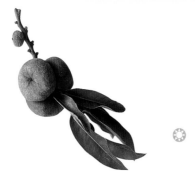

E ʻAI I KA MEA I LOAʻA.

What you have, eat.
(Be satisfied with what you have.)
—Mary Kawena Pukui

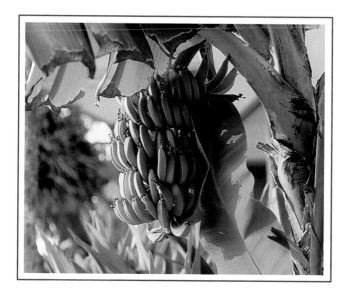

83

"For Hawaiian people, hospitality
(ho'okipa) is a way of life. My grandmother
always called out to strangers to come in and rest,
eat and drink before continuing their journey.
That is the Hawaiian way, that is the spirit of
aloha. Even though my grandparents did not have
much, that was the custom—you never turn
anybody away. No matter what you have, you
always offer to share. You never hoard or hide,
you never turn away anyone in need. In old
Hawai'i, you may eventually find that the one
you did not offer hospitality to was a
Hawaiian deity in the guise of a mortal."

Daniel Akaka, Cultural Adviser, Island of Hawai'i

E HEA I KE KANAKA E KOMO MALOKO
E HĀNAI AI A HEWA KA WAHA.

**Call to the person to enter; feed him
until he can take no more.**
—Mary Kawena Pukui

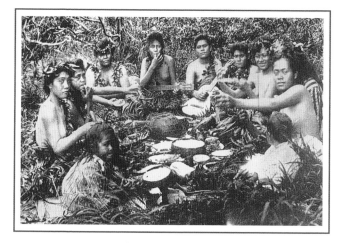

Hawaiians have reverence for every part of nature from the oceans and mountains, to trees, flowers, rocks, wind, rain, fire, sky, stars, sun and moon. They believe there is mana (spiritual power or energy) in all and this mana can be tapped by people for strength. Just sitting with nature and becoming part of nature can heal. Each of the Hawaiian Islands resonates its own personality, from the oldest, nurturing motherly Island of Kaua'i to the youngest Island of Hawai'i. It follows that each island's salts, clays and plants used in healing preparations are believed to take on the characteristics of the island. The Island of Hawai'i draws thousands of people each year for healing. It is considered the island of renewal because it is still rebirthing, pouring lava into the ocean daily. This is seen as sacred and powerful energy.

ĒWE HĀNAU O KA ʻĀINA.

Natives of the land.
—Mary Kawena Pukui

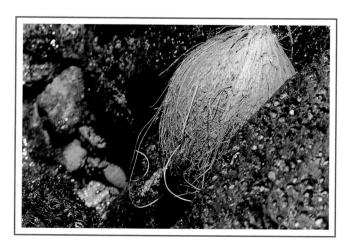

"Know that man is not superior
to our earth. Know we are stewards of the
land and the ocean. Aloha is to share, to give and
to receive. The sunlight and the moonlight are our
source of energy. We need to know those things
are important to us. The importance has to
be every day, all of the time."

Anonymous, Hawaiian Guide, Island of Hawai'i

HE ALI'I KA 'ĀINA; HE KAUWĀ KE KANAKA.

The land is a chief; man is its servant.
—Mary Kawena Pukui

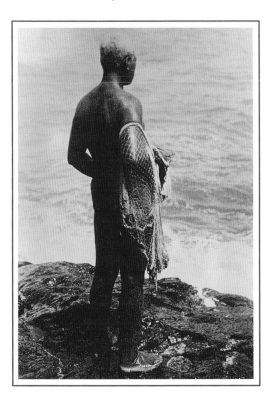

Even in death forgiveness is crucial for the journey onward.

"When my father died my brother
gave the eulogy. He displayed a rock and two kī
(ti) leaves. He asked if our father had offended
anyone, to please forgive him by putting that
thought into this rock. Also, if anyone had
offended him to do the same. He will then wrap
the rock in the kī (ti) leaves and drop it
in the deepest depth of the ocean and
let it be forgotten forever."

Kupuna Alapaʻi Kahuʻena, Lāʻau Lapaʻau
(Herbal Practitioner), Oʻahu

HAʻALELE I KA LĀ KA MEA MAHANA.

Has left the warmth of the sun (died).
—Mary Kawena Pukui

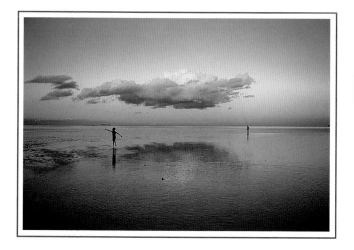

When westerners arrived, traditional Hawaiian healing was banned. It is only recently massage, herbal medicine, spiritual chanting and hula have been practiced and taught openly. Still today traditional Hawaiian healers are banned from treating their own family in many modern health clinics. It is hard to believe earth-based healing practices used for more than a thousand years are dubbed "alternative" while synthetic chemicals, cutting the body open and cutting off limbs, burning the body with radiation and undergoing mind-altering drug treatments is acceptable as modern medicine (less than a hundred years old). Hawaiian healers believe in cures, not treatments and you do not need medical insurance. All the ʻāina offers is free to those who need healing. Many healers I spoke with trust in the prediction of their ancestors— that when the time is right, their healing and traditions will be asked for again. I believe they will be revered.

HE KOʻE KA PULE A KAHUNA,
HE MOE NO A ʻONI MAI.

**The prayer of a kahuna is like a worm;
it may lie dormant but it will wriggle along.**
—Mary Kawena Pukui

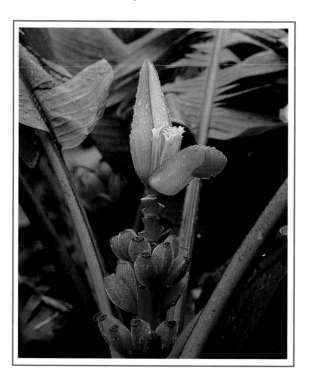

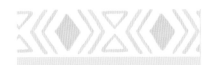

"In Hawaiian there is an aloha expression
my grandfather used as a reminder that all things
are always in rightness—right place, right time,
right being. This is known as 'I ka pono mea.'
One of five universal laws (Nā Kānāwai Aʻo
Holoʻokoʻa) is Kānāwai Mōakaaka which
translates as the smiling law. This resonated with
Hawaiians because they understood the universe is
in place to serve us and does so smilingly. With
this in mind grandfather would always say 'choose
only thoughts of aloha to have aloha experiences
and if in the moment you cannot think aloha,
then no think at all'! One soon learned the
importance of choice—pono (excellence,
rightness) or pilikia (trauma, drama)…
and once that choice was made, the
experience of likeness followed."

Mahealani Kuamoʻo-Henry, Kumu ʻElele o nā Kūpuna
(teacher messenger for the ancestors), Island of Hawaiʻi

ʻO HAWAIʻI KUʻU ʻĀINA ALOHA.

Hawaiʻi my beloved land.
—Mary Kawena Pukui

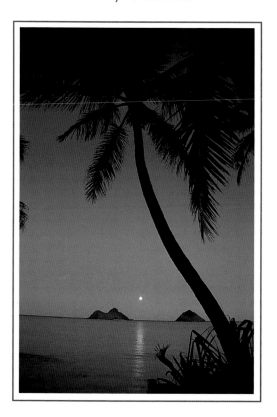

PHOTO CREDITS

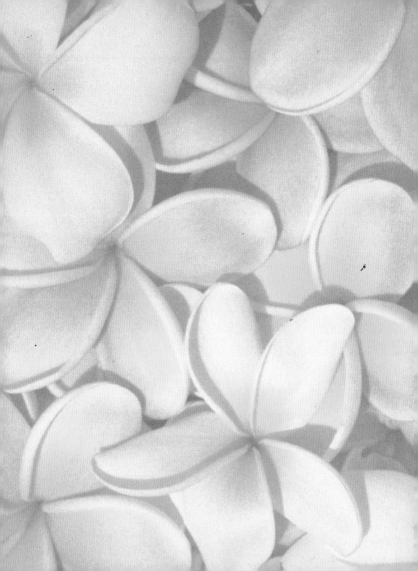